If Your Dog is Fat

You're Not Getting Enough Exercise!

How to Lose 15 Pounds in 30 Minutes

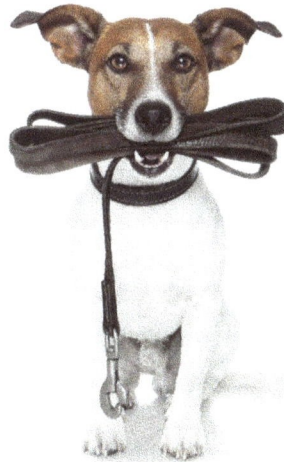

Patricia A. Brill, PhD

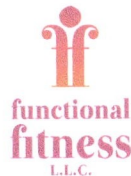

functional fitness
L.L.C.

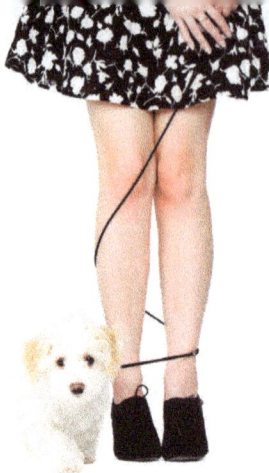

If Your Dog Is Fat You're Not Getting Enough Exercise!

© 2013 by Patricia A. Brill

Published by Functional Fitness L.L.C.

ISBN-13: 978-0-9815551-2-6 (paperback)

Printed in America

Cover art: © istockphoto.com/damedeeso. Pages: ©iStock/mimic51 (page ii), Kim Hartz Photography (page iii), ©iStock/PK-Photos (page iv), ©iStock/PK-Photos (page vi), ©PhotoExpress/maumau-design (page 4), ©iStock/Vivienstock (page 5), ©iStock/Sadeugra (page 7), ©iStock/fokusgood (page 9), ©iStock/stray_cat (page 11), ©iStock/Nikada (page 12), ©PhotoExpress/Pixel Memoirs (page 13), ©Fotolia/K.-U. HaBler (page 15), ©iStock/temele (page 16), ©iStock/ruthrose (page 17), ©iStock/Ljupco (page 18), ©iStock/irin717 (page 19), PhotoExpress/Fauna & Flora (page 21), ©PhotoExpress/devilpup (page 22), ©PhotoExpress/Clint Haimerl (page 23), ©iStock/DPLight (page 24), ©iStock/Mlenny (page 30) ©PhotoExpress/Marco Antonio Fdez (page 32).

Book design by DesignForBooks.com

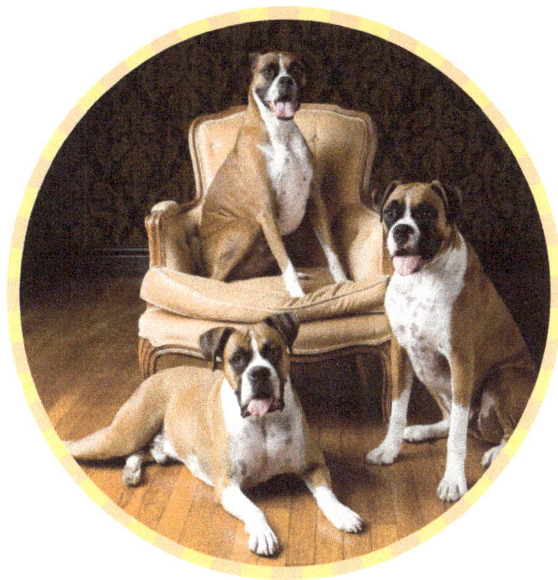

Dear Mom,

The happiest day of our life was when you walked into the pound, came right up to our cage, and said, "I want to adopt these dogs." Our tails were wagging so fast we couldn't stop them. We want to thank you for adopting us. By your act of kindness, you have made such a difference in our lives. We are safe, happy, healthy and the best of friends. We have a great life! Now we want to help you. You haven't been home as much lately and have been working very hard. You look stressed! So, we want to return the favor, totally unselfishly, and we want to take you for a walk every day. This way, you can catch up on quality time with us and feel a whole lot better, too.

Love

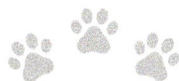

Turbo, Boxster, and Cayman

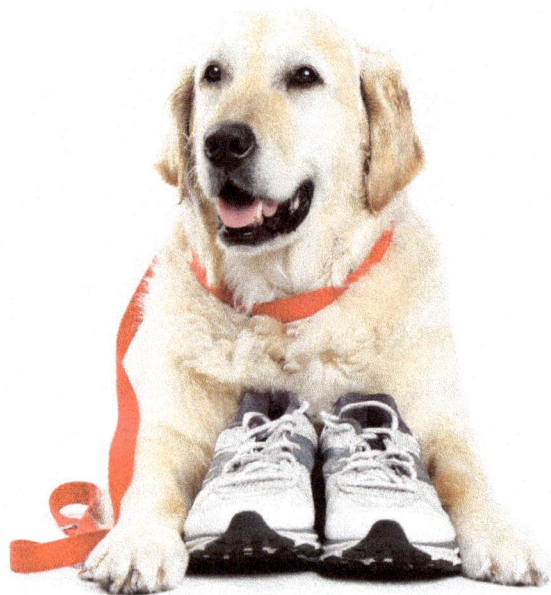

Contents

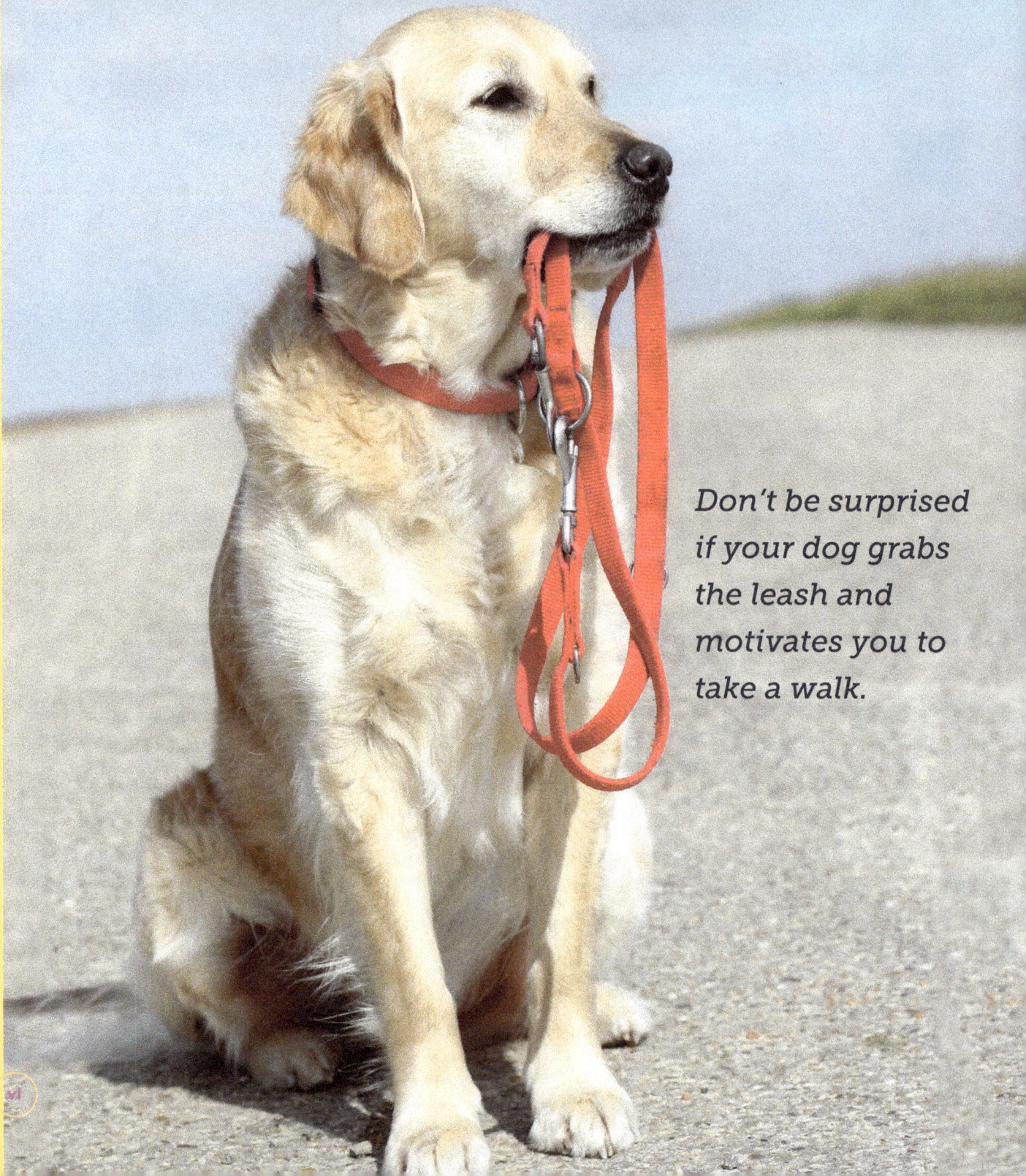

Don't be surprised if your dog grabs the leash and motivates you to take a walk.

Get a New Leash on Life

He is your friend, your partner, your defender, your dog. You are his life, his love, his leader. He will be yours, faithful and true, to the last beat of his heart. You owe it to him to be worthy of such devotion.

—*Unknown*

Fewer than one half of all adults in the United States engage in recommended levels of physical activity, and nearly 25 percent of adults do not participate in any leisure-time physical activity. An estimated 25% to 40% of dogs in the US are also overweight or obese. Inactivity has been shown to be a significant risk factor for obesity in dogs as well as in humans. Dogs gain weight for the same reason that people do—they eat more calories than they expend throughout the day.

Dog walking is a purposeful, physical activity that can have health benefits for humans as well as canines. Walking a dog can contribute to a physically active lifestyle for you and your dog. In addition, walking with your dog will help you have a positive outlook on life, a renewed interest in being active, and increased levels of happiness.

Here are some other benefits that can occur from walking your dog on a regular basis:

- Boost energy
- Improve balance
- Keep joints flexible
- Help obtain healthy weight
- Feel better—personal fulfillment
- Strengthen and tone your muscles
- Contribute to a physically active lifestyle
- Strengthen bond between you and your dog
- Increased social interaction—meet your neighbors

Could man's best friend help you obtain your optimal weight, reduce stress, and improve your health and well-being? You bet they can. Studies have shown that dog owners who walk their dogs on a regular basis are more physically active than non-dog owners, or owners who do not walk their dogs. The American College of Sports Medicine (ACSM) and the American Heart Association released new recommendations on the quantity and quality of exercise for adults. They should get at least 150 minutes of moderate-intensity exercise per week.

This recommendation is also in accordance with The Humane Society. They recommend for optimal health and fitness, dogs should be walked twice daily, at least 15 minutes per walk.

The Return on Investment (ROI) can be enormous for as little as the cost of a leash and a good pair of walking shoes. So give it a try. You'll be surprised how good you will feel! And when you feel good, you'll be prone to make healthier choices for you and your dog.

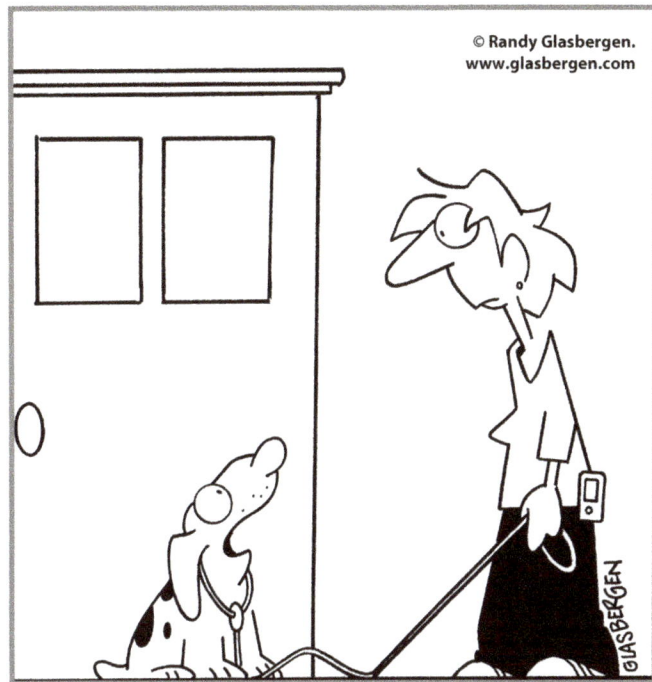

© Randy Glasbergen.
www.glasbergen.com

"How come you need $150 walking shoes, but I have to do 2 miles in bare feet?!"

After a while, your dog will make walking a part of their daily routine. They can serve as a great motivator to get more exercise. Just think, you can always teach them to fetch your walking shoes.

If you practice healthy behaviors 80%—90% of the time it won't matter if you "stray" the other 10%—20%.

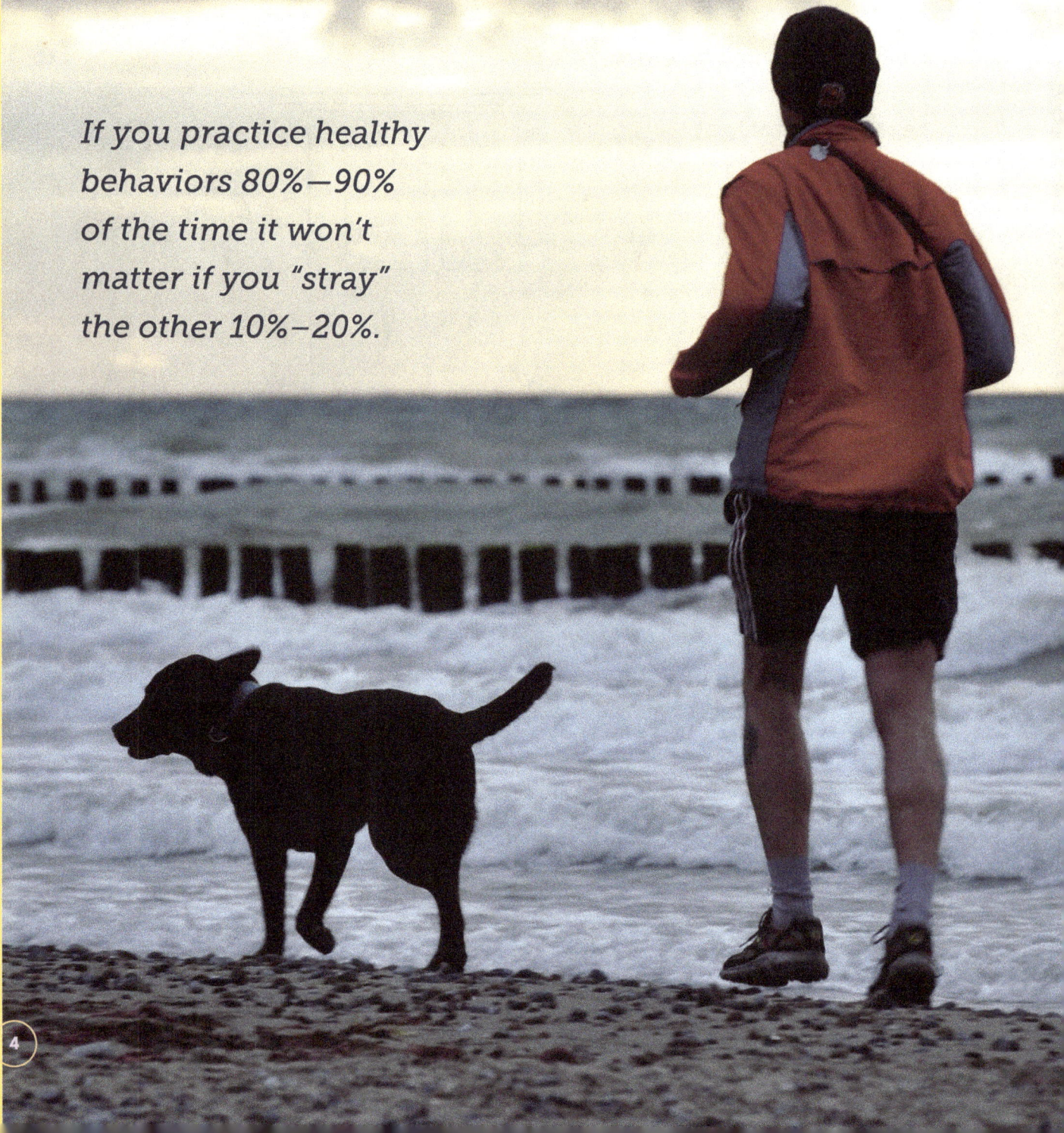

What You Think About You Bring About

Whatever the mind can conceive
and believe, it can achieve!

—*Napoleon Hill*

Behavior Change is basically taking an unhealthy behavior (for example lack of physical activity) and replacing it with a healthy behavior (like walking your dog). Everyone knows they should be active throughout the day. However knowing and doing are two separate things. I have a "bone" of contention with the expression "Knowledge is Power". Knowledge is not enough to make you make a change in your lifestyle, "Acting" on knowledge is what will result in power. Everyone knows that eating healthy foods, exercising on a regular basis, getting eight hours of sleep, and reducing the stressors in our life will help us live a long, healthy, fit life. But how many of us really make this a priority in our life by taking action to change it?

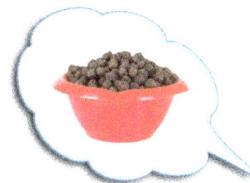

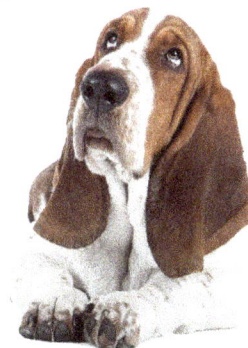

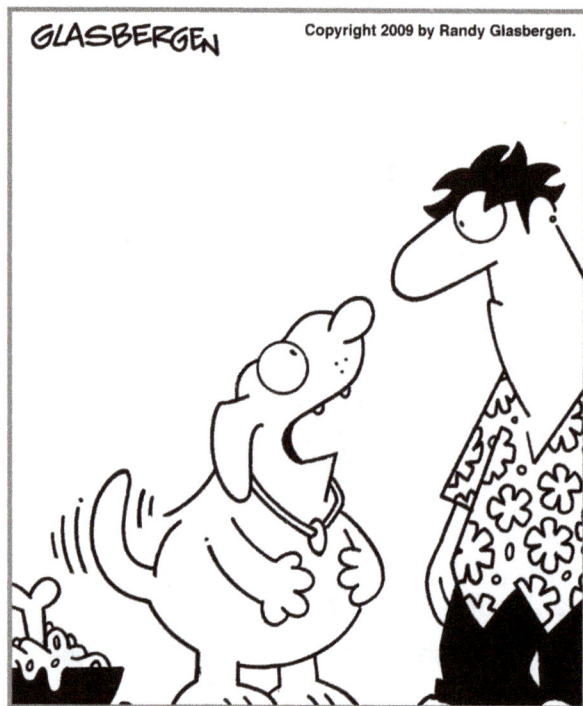

GLASBERGEN

Copyright 2009 by Randy Glasbergen.

"I don't understand how I got so fat! Doesn't tail wagging count as cardio?"

Have you heard about the law of attraction—what you think about you bring about. Well I'm here to tell you it really works. For most of us however, it works in a negative way. We tend to focus over and over on the negative things in our lives. I'm overweight, I'm tired, and I'm stressed. However it is possible to maximize your health benefits by staying in a positive state of mind. Positive thinking can help you focus on what you want and bring about the changes you want to see.

What do you think is the one thing that separates those who obtain their goal from those who do not—"*Action*." Jack Canfield (Chicken Soup for the Soul) says taking action is ultimately your decision, so act in ways that produce more of what you want. People who get results get it through Attr-"Action." They are attracting the positive action or result they want. So if you want to obtain a healthy weight, reduce stress, reduce your risk for chronic disease, or feel good about yourself, then make an active lifestyle a priority in your life and take action.

2 French Fries Weigh 40 Pounds

Properly trained, a man can be a dog's best friend

—*Corey Ford*

I know you've heard the adage, "You are what you eat". Well here is an example that really puts it into perspective, at least for me. Matthew Bennett, author of *FAT MATT, Because Whining Doesn't Burn Calories* (*www.fatmatt.com*) developed a scenario where eating just two French fries a day could cause you to gain forty pounds over ten years. Here's how it goes.

Putting on 40 pounds over ten years means gaining an average of 4 pounds per year:

> (40 pounds divided by 10 years = 4 pounds per year) That's .33 (one-third) pound per month: (4 pounds divided by 12 months = .33 (one-third) of a pound per month).

Or approximately .01 (one one-hundredth) of a pound per day: (.33 pounds divided by 30 days). Since one pound of stored fat represents

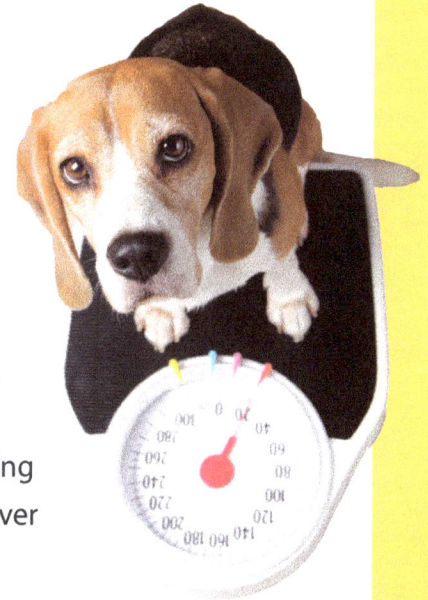

about 3500 calories to your body, and since $3500 \times .01 = 35$, to achieve the feat of gaining 40 pounds in ten years, you simply have to consume a whopping 35 extra calories every day! That's the equivalent of half a slice of bread, three Lifesavers, or two hefty French fries! This should make you think next time you want a snack.

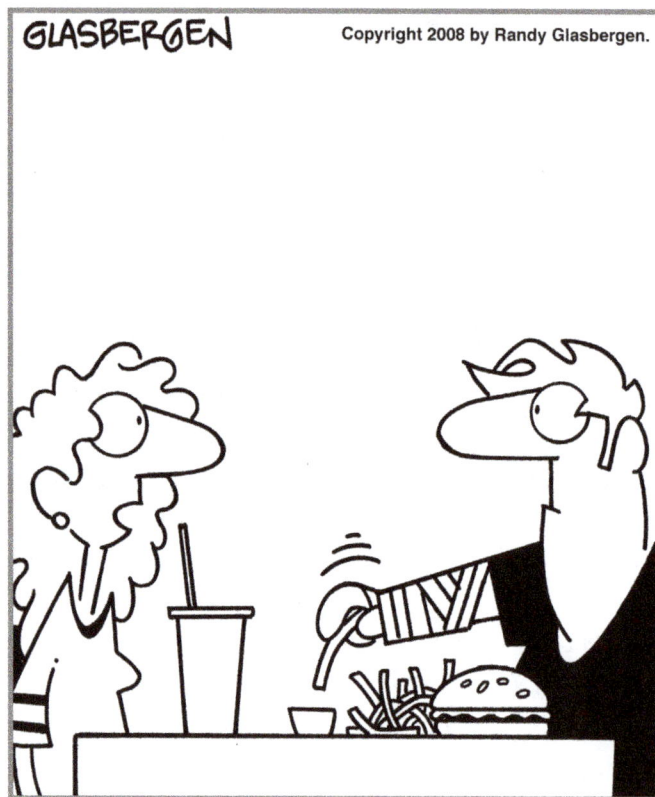

"You know it's time to improve your diet when you get carpel tunnel from dipping french fries in ketchup!"

Let Sleeping Dogs Lie

You can run with the big dogs or
sit on the porch and bark

—*Wallace Arnold*

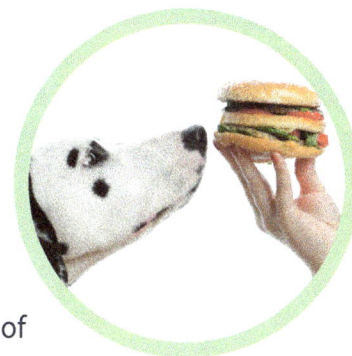

Do you ever over eat because you are bored? Actually any type of emotion, happy, sad, fear, depression, or excitement will cause people to over eat, but boredom is the worse. Boredom can be a major contributing factor toward obesity in your dog as well. How many couches, tables, shoes, slippers, or other personal items have been chewed or destroyed because your dogs were bored? Sedentary dogs tend to get into trouble if left alone with nothing to do. Like humans, dogs will eat out of boredom if food is available. If they are well exercised, they tend to sleep while you are away and the furniture is safe. I guess the adage "Move it or Lose it" holds true for dogs as well. If you don't exercise your dog, you will lose something of value. Exercise on a regular basis can help alleviate the boredom and collateral damage. Now I can fully understand that a dog left home alone all day

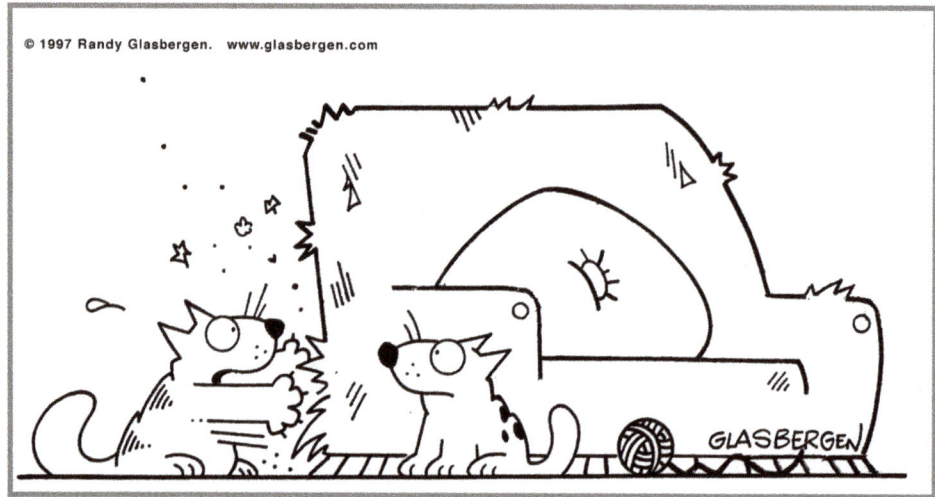

© 1997 Randy Glasbergen. www.glasbergen.com

GLASBERGEN

"This exercise is great for your arms, shoulders, chest and back. Do four sets of 15 repetitions, then move on to the yarn ball for your aerobics"

may get bored and destroy something. In theory, if there are two or three dogs left in the house alone, they shouldn't be bored. They have someone to play with. So I thought.

One afternoon my husband and I left the house for less than an hour. As soon as Turbo, Boxster, and Cayman, our three boxers (named after Porsches) saw us back out of the driveway, they jumped off the couch, grabbed their 4' x 4' doggie bed, drug it through the kitchen, and then pulled the bed out the doggie door into the back yard. I can see them now, pulling and tugging, tugging and pulling, ripping the bed apart until foam is scattered all over the back yard. I'm sure it looked like it snowed in July. We had no idea this was going on until John our next door neighbor called us and said, "I think the dogs are into something they shouldn't be." In case you are wondering, did John come over and stop them from destroying the bed further? No, he took pictures! Thanks John!

So, to prevent your dog from overeating, putting on extra weight, and destroying your pillows, push back from the table, pick up the dog food dish, and take your dog on a walk!

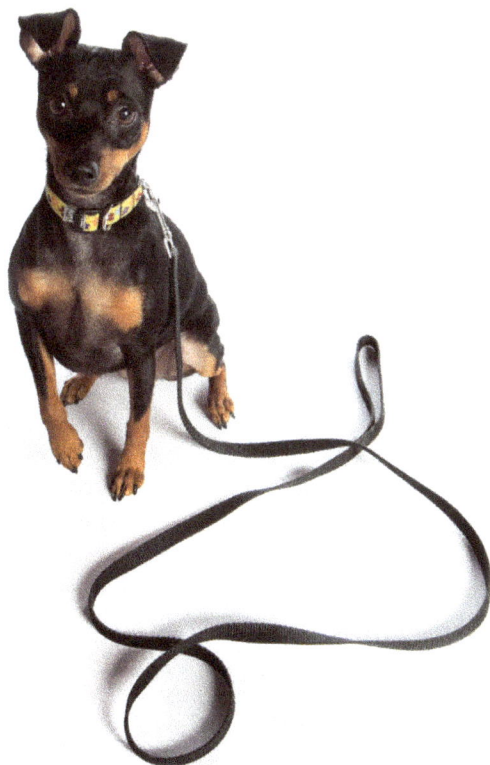

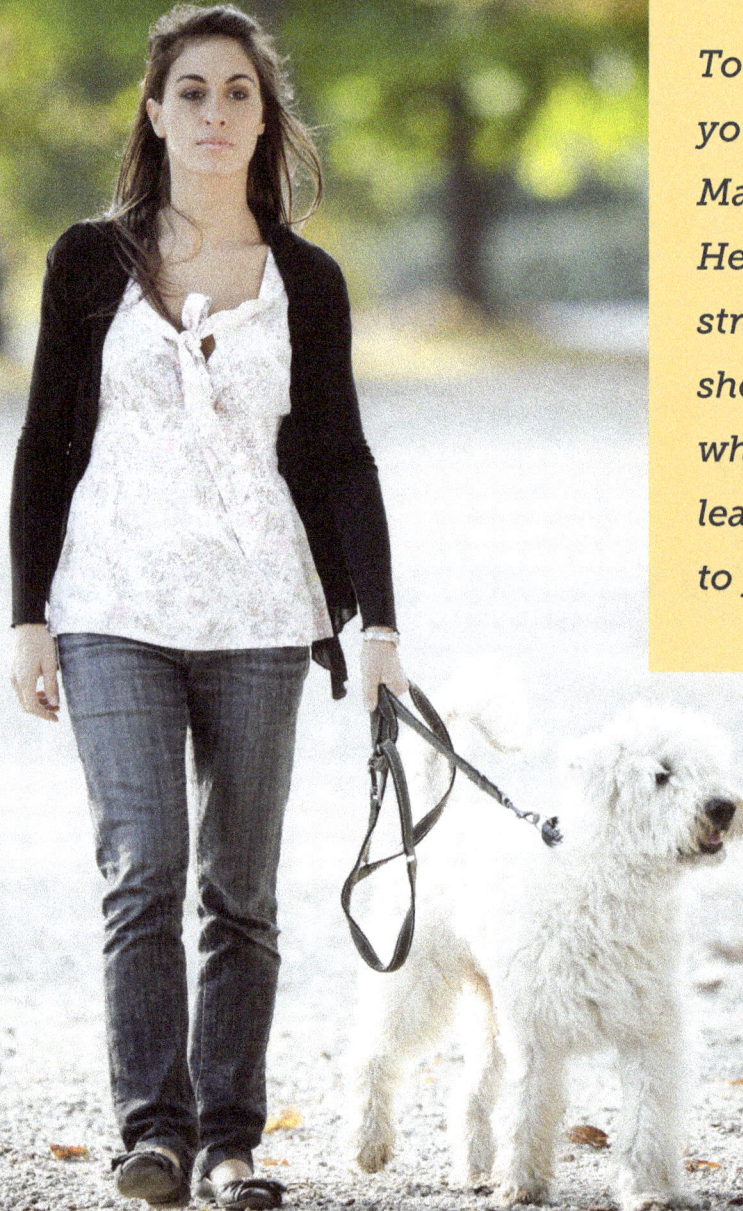

To get the most out of your walk with your dog: Maintain good posture— Head up, spine back, look straight ahead. Arms and shoulders should be loose while holding onto the leash. Keep your dog next to your side.

How to Lose 15 Pounds in 30 minutes

If walking is man's best medicine (Hippocrates), and
A dog is man's best friend (Unknown), then . . .
Walking man's best friend must be man's
best medicine for a healthy life

—*P.A. Brill*

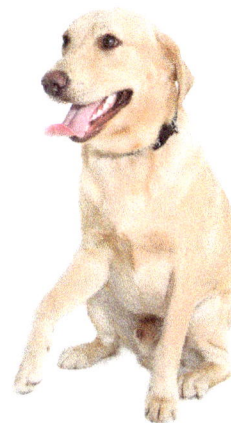

Here's a positive way to think about calories rather than the calories in the 2 French Fries scenario. (And who could only eat just two fries anyways?) For example, on average you expend 200 calories walking 30 minutes. So walking 30 minutes a day for 5 days equals 1000 calories.

If you walk five days a week for 52 weeks, you then will have expended 52,000 calories. Remember from the French Fry example in Chapter 3, one pound is equal to 3500 calories. So 52,000 divided by 3500 equals approximately 15 pounds lost in one year. Disclaimer . . . This is just a rough estimate. However, you get the point. Expending extra

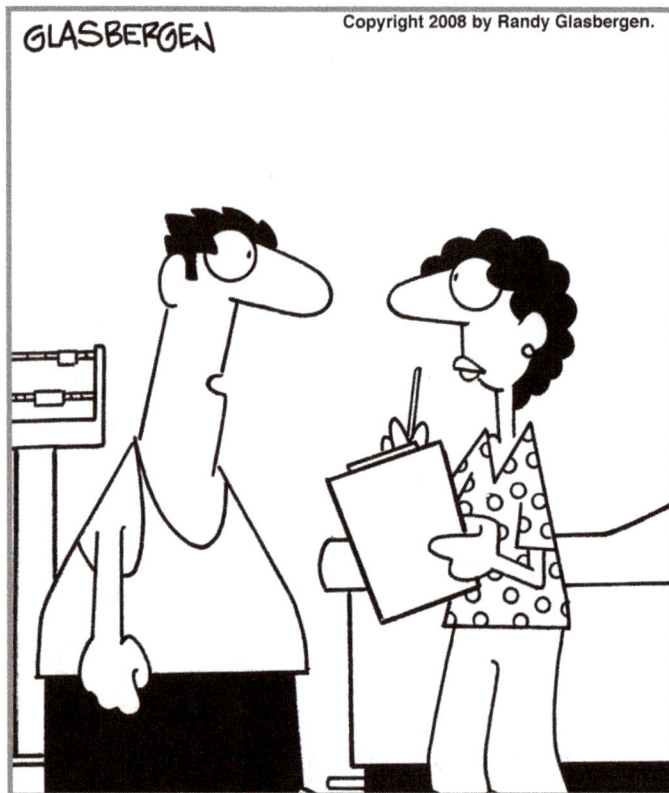

"I must be eating right. I'm narrow at the top and wide at the bottom, just like the Food Pyramid!"

calories over time will result in weight loss. The bottom line is that walking your dog is an excellent way to expend calories to help you achieve an optimum weight for both you and your dog.

If you or your dogs are new to walking, go slow at first. Start with short periods of activity such as a 10 minute walk a day, and then gradually increase the time to 30 minutes a day, most days of the week. If you can't fit in 30 minutes a day all at one time, divide the walks into two, fifteen minute walks. You will still meet the American College of Sports Medicine and The Humane Society's recommendation for 30 minutes of moderate exercise most days of the week. Over time, and as your overall fitness level improves, gradually increase the speed and distance of your walks. As always, before trying any new rigorous exercise routine, consult your health care provider as well as your veterinarian.

But don't just stop at 30 minutes a day. Look for more opportunities to take your dog for a walk, even if it is just to the mailbox and back. This is a great way to give you and your dog more exercise, which means more calories burned, which means more weight loss.

•

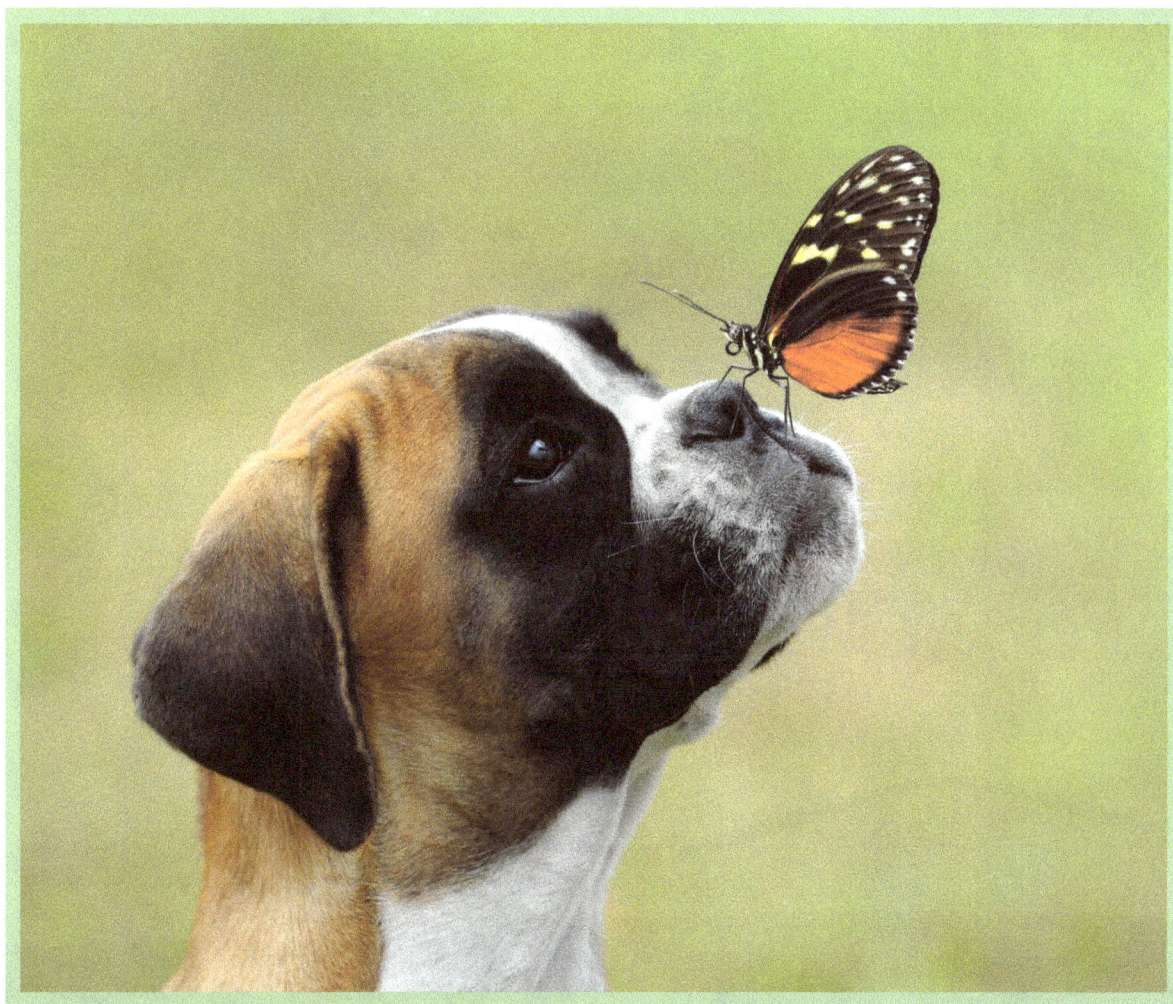

If in doubt about your dog's health and readiness to walk, take him to the vet. And likewise, before you start on a new walking program, consult with your healthcare provider as well.

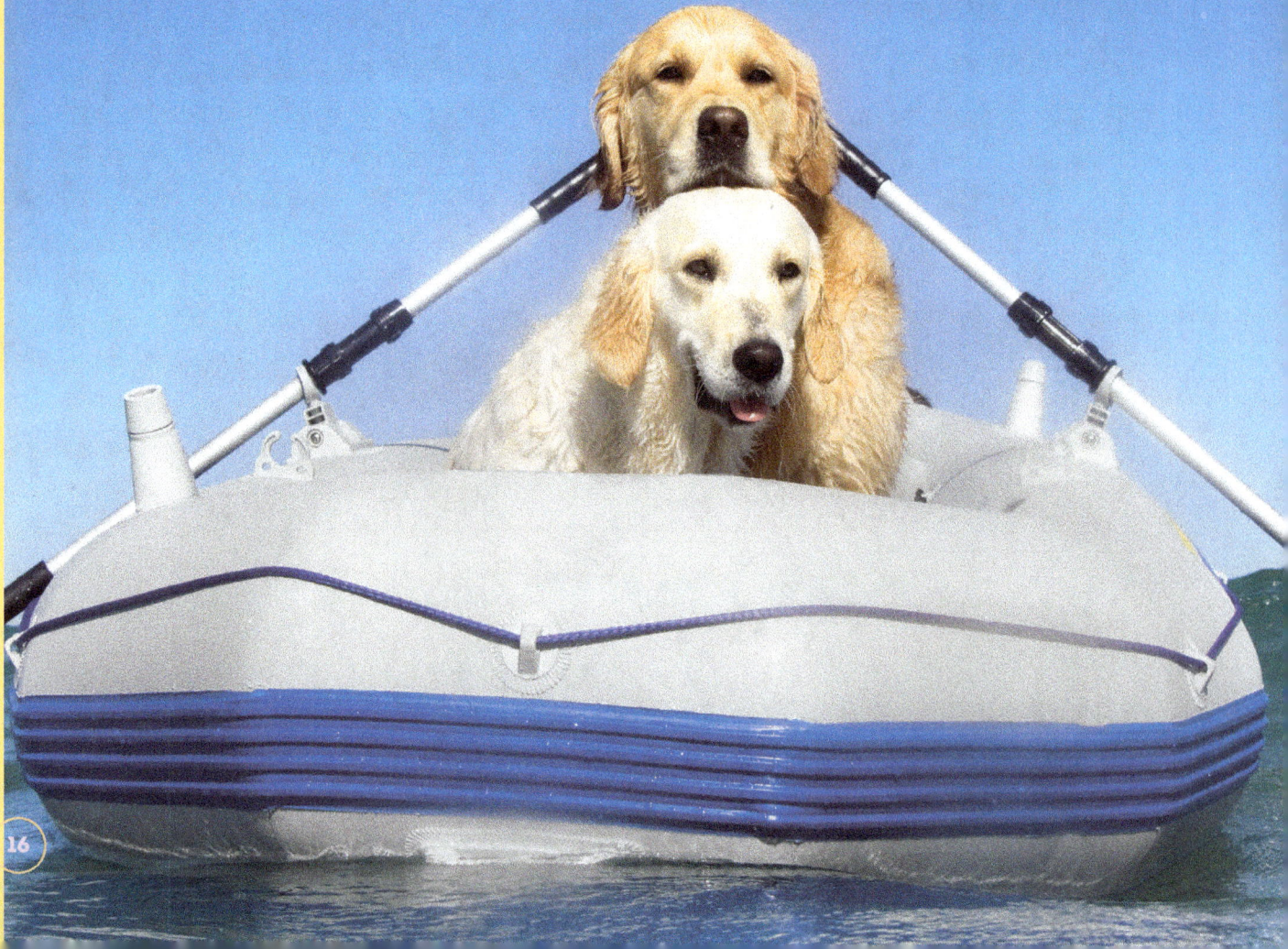

Fire Hydrant Training Program

Never stand between a dog and the hydrant

— *John Peers*

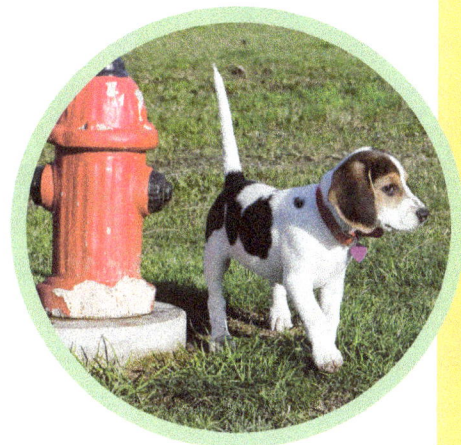

If you find yourself at a point where you are not losing weight like you first did when you started walking your dog, vary the intensity of your walk. You will become more efficient at burning fat than walking at a steady pace. To help you vary the intensity of your walk, try the Fire Hydrant Training program. Find a walking route that has fire hydrants along it. Most streets have hydrants placed approximately 100 feet apart. Walk at your regular pace from the first fire hydrant to the second. When you get to the second fire hydrant, pick up the pace until you get to the next hydrant. Resume your regular pace until the next hydrant. Continue on throughout your walk.

Remember in the Introduction section of this book we said that we need to walk at a moderate pace (brisk walk) for health benefits. Well,

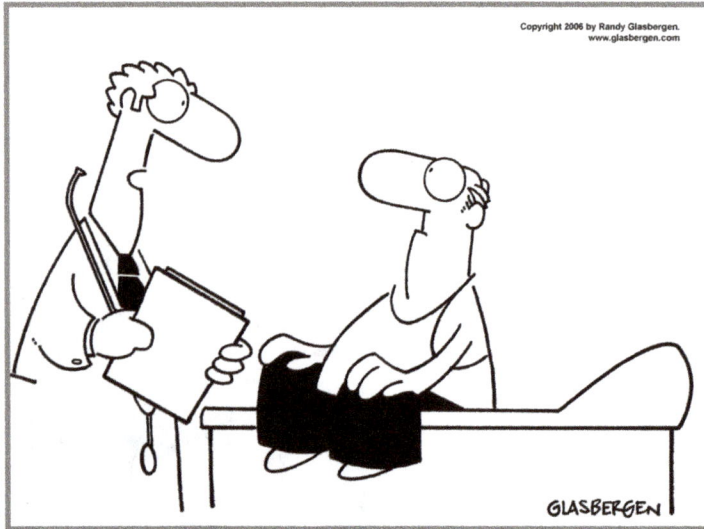

"Spend more time outside with your dog. Teach him how to throw a stick for you to chase."

larger dogs can help us pick up the pace.

If you are thinking about jogging, only jog with your dog if they are fit and at an optimum weight. If you do start jogging, gradually build up to a greater distance each week. Check with your vet before putting your dog on a jogging program.

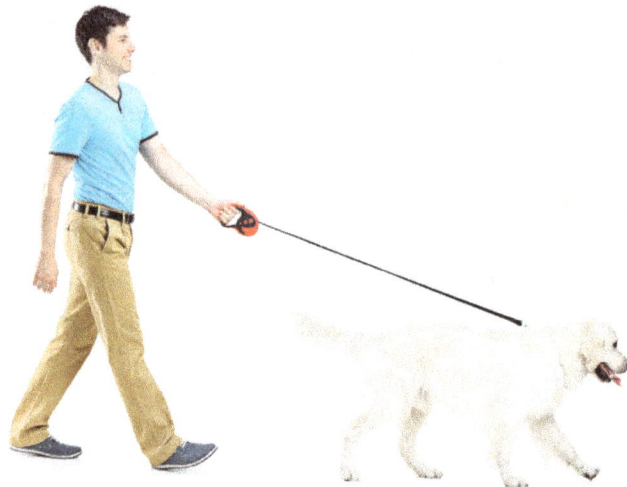

Strength Training—You May be Barking up the Wrong Tree

Dogs are not only our whole lives,
but they make our lives whole.

—*Roger Caras*

Traditional strength training exercises such as the biceps curl, the sit up, or the leg extension can easily be performed on machines at your local health club or at home using dumbbells or resistance bands. What a lot of people don't realize is that these traditional strength exercises are training isolated joints and muscles. This training is adequate for building muscle; however it does not train the body to meet the specific demands of daily life. So, to meet the demands of "daily life", you need to be functionally fit.

So what is functional fitness you ask? Functional fitness not only includes cardiovascular fitness, but it also includes other fitness components such as: Muscular Strength, Muscular Endurance,

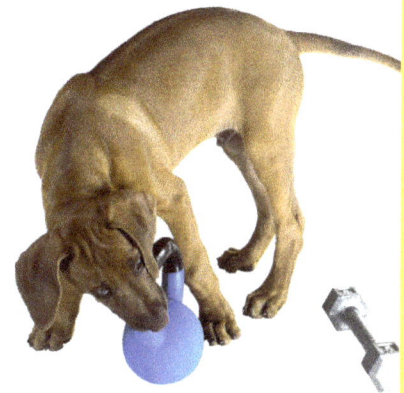

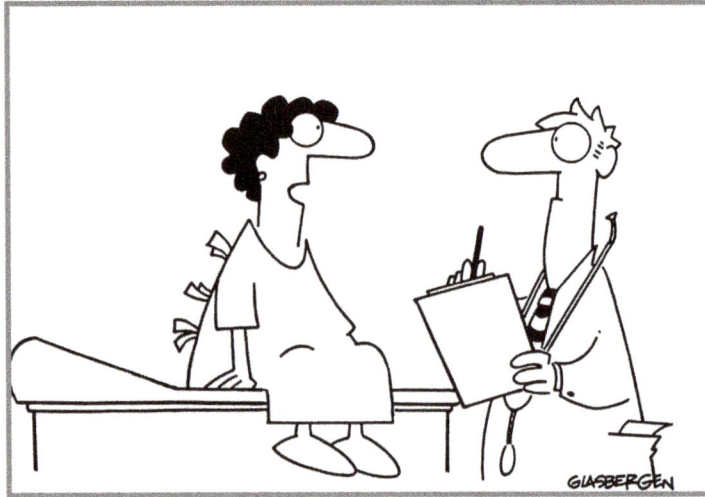

"Drink lots of water if I want to lose weight? My dog drinks from the toilet all day and he weighs a ton."

Balance, Flexibility, and Range of Motion. Muscular Endurance comes into play when you are taking long walks down the beach with your dog. Flexibility is needed to pass the leash from one hand to the other behind your back when your dog decides to run around you. Balance is needed when you are walking 2 or more dogs at a time and they want to go in opposite directions. And most importantly, muscular strength is needed to keep your dog from chasing another dog down the street, or when you have to carry your dog in a cage to the vets' office.

Performing functional training exercises is also a good way to burn fat. These exercises increase the amount of muscle mass used in the exercises. The number of calories burned is directly related to how much muscle is stimulated during training: more muscle equates to a greater caloric expenditure. Functional training allows you to get more out of your workouts by combining moves that can help you burn more calories, engage more muscles and joints, and save you time.

Included with this book is an exercise program designed specifically for you. *A New Leash on Life* program focuses on movement patterns used in walking and taking care of your dog, as well as many other daily tasks. Performing this program on a regular basis will strengthen your arms, shoulders, abdomen, legs, buttocks, and lower back.

If you already exercise, start out with 2–5 pound dumbbells for women and 5–10 pound dumbbells for men. As the exercises get easier, increase the weight of the dumbbells by small increments.

If you are new to exercising, I would recommend you forget about using weights entirely at first. Your first step should be to teach your body to control and balance its own weight as well as work on your form. Once you can control and balance your own body weight, then you can start working with added weights.

Some of the best lower body exercises for you are squats and lunges. These exercises are one of the most basic and functional movements that you can perform for accomplishing a variety of daily tasks. Not only do squats work the entire lower body in one movement, they also mimic movements we do all day long. When you combine upper body exercises with squats or lunges, you've got a more effective, time efficient, functional training program you can perform with ease.

While bodybuilding is for aesthetics and power lifting is for performance, functional training is for building a person's strength, balance, and endurance to meet the demands of daily living.

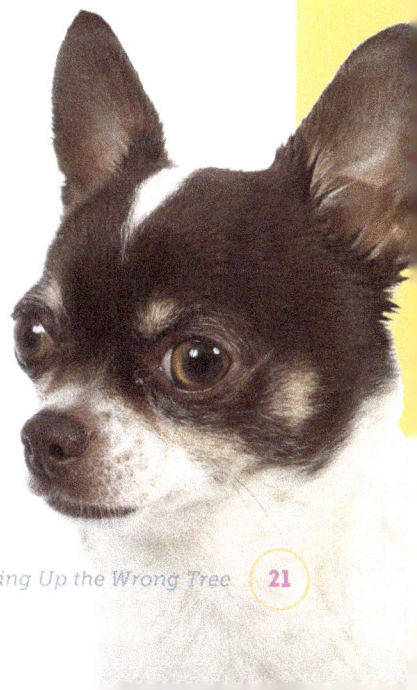

Your dog can actually be the most reliable exercise partner you've ever had.

Walking Safety Tips for your Dog

- Start slow, especially if your dog is out of shape. Keep walks under 10–15 minutes the first week. Over time, gradually take longer, brisker walks.

- Watch your dog. Stop if your dog shows signs of limping or trouble breathing, or is falling behind. If your dog wants to stop, don't force her to keep going.

- Make sure your dog is wearing a collar and current ID tag and/or license.

- Always walk your dog on a leash, however avoid extended leashes.

- If you walk your dog at night, dress in light colors and put reflectors on your dog as well as yourself.

- Keep feeding and exercise separate. Taking your dog out for a walk shortly after a meal could cause bloat which could become a life-threatening condition.

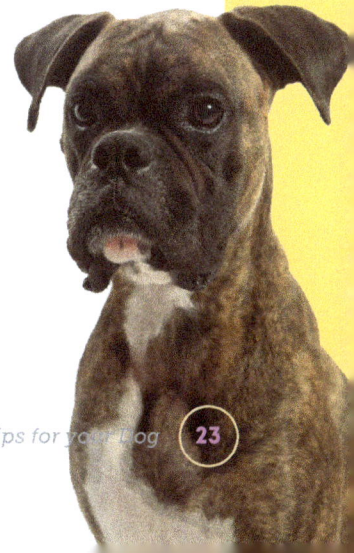

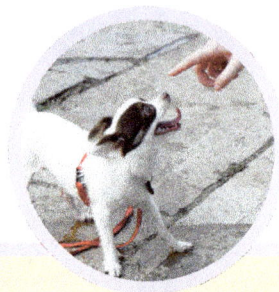

How to teach your dog to heel

🐾 The proper way to walk a dog is with the dog on your left side, and the leash across in front of you, held in your right hand.

🐾 The dog should walk with his head or shoulder even with your hip at will. You are not holding the leash tight to keep your dog in place. The leash is slack between you, with no contact.

🐾 Walk at a decent pace, with your shoulders up. Walk confidently and proud, because dogs can sense lack of confidence or tension.

🐾 Make sure your dog gets plenty of water before, during, and after your walk—at any time of year.

Hot Weather

🐾 Avoid walking midday in sunny weather when the temperature is at its hottest. Schedule walks for early morning or in the evening.

🐾 Walk your dog in grassy areas or on dirt paths. Paved roads can be too hot for your dog's paws.

🐾 Look for signs of overheating such as excessive panting, difficulty breathing, drooling, weakness, or stupor.

🐾 Avoid unknown lawns or landscaped areas that may contain fertilizers and pesticides.

Cold Weather

🐾 Road salt and ice melted chemicals can also injure your dog's paws or be toxic if ingested, so wipe his paws when you return home.

"New Leash on Life" Exercise Program

Your Walking Plan

Set realistic goals for you and your dog each week—Start slowly, progress gradually. Strive to meet the American College of Sports Medicine and the American Heart Association's recommendations for adults:

- 2 hours 30 min (150 min) week / 30 minutes a day—5 days a week.

- Moderate intensity aerobic activity—walk at a brisk pace.

- Or 10 minutes at a time, 3 times a day.

For greatest health benefits:

- 5 hours (300 min) week / approx. 45 minutes a day.

- And . . . Perform the "A New Leash on Life" program 2+ days a week

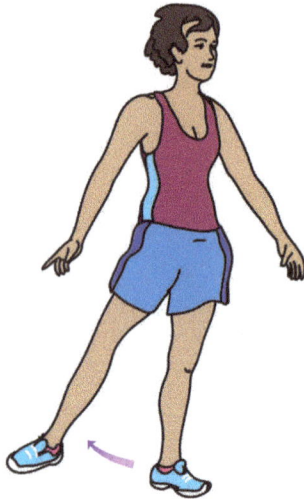

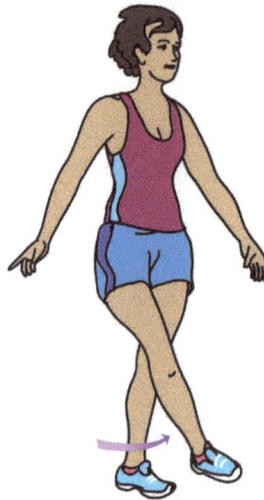

1

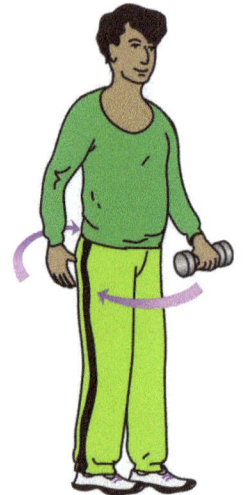

2

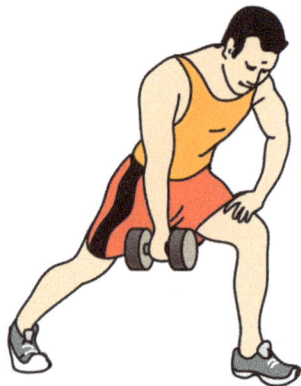

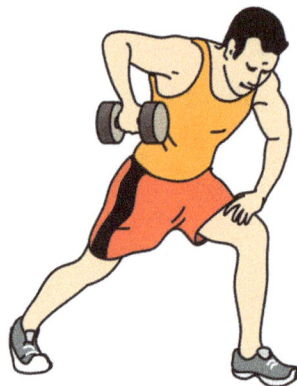

5

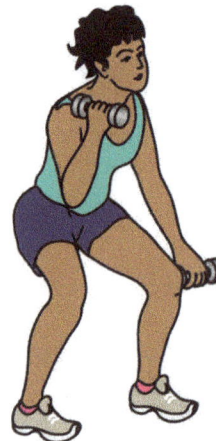

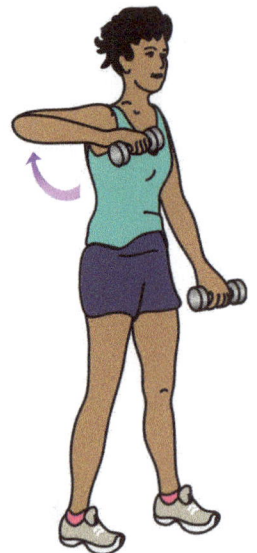

6

See instructions on pages 28–29.

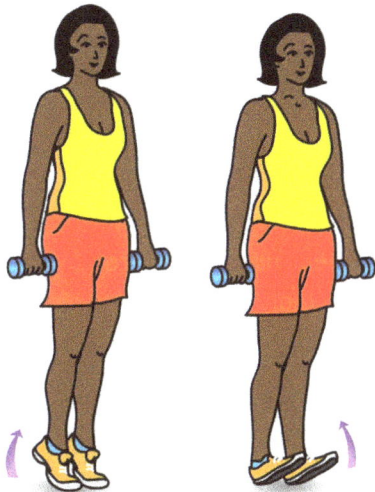

3

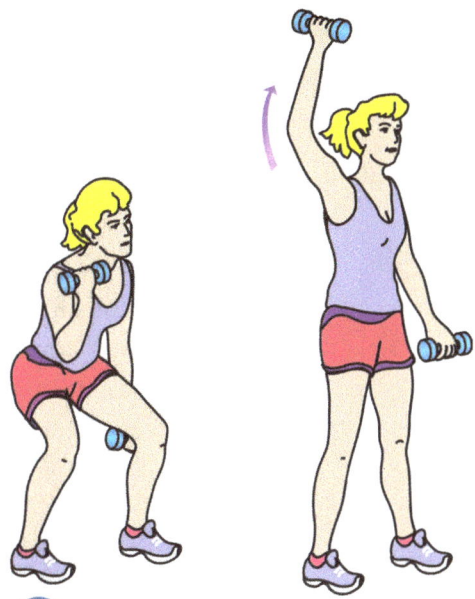

4

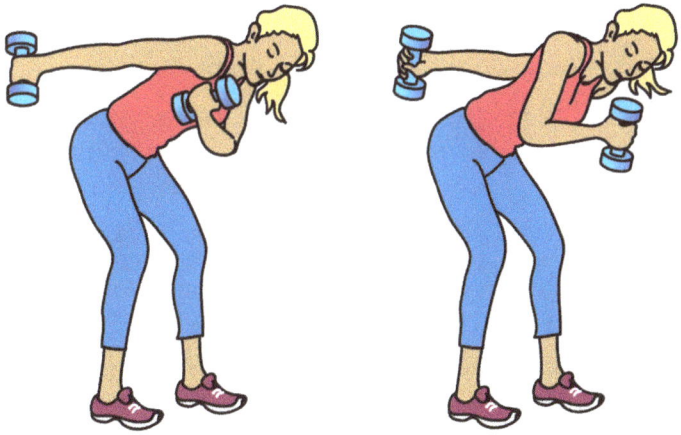

7

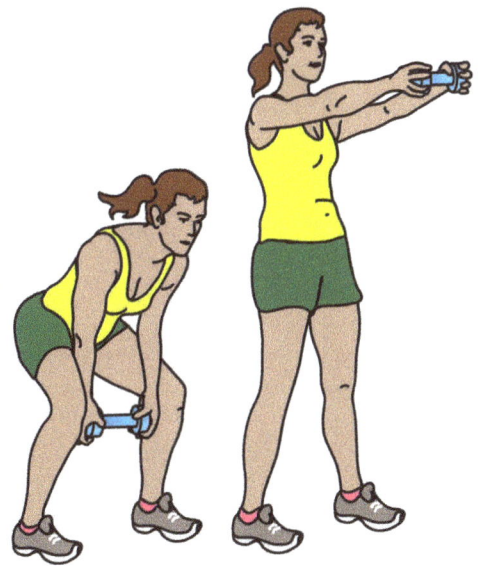

8

1 Leg to Side & Cross

Stand with feet shoulder with apart. Keeping the back straight, slowly raise the right leg out to the side away from the body (Approx. 1 ft.). Hold 3 seconds. Slowly cross leg in front of body. Hold 3 seconds. Return to starting position. Perform 8 to 12 repetitions. Switch legs. Perform 8 to 12 repetitions with the left leg.

2 Dumbbell Pass

Slowly pass the dumbbell around the waist 8 to 12 times. Stop. Reverse direction 8 to 12 times. Repeat series 2 times.

3 Heel/Toe Raise

Hold a dumbbell in one hand. Slowly rise up on the toes. Hold 3 seconds. Slowly roll back on the heels. Repeat 8 to 12 times.

4 One Arm Push-Up

Holding a dumbbell in the right hand with the palm facing the right shoulder, sit back into a squat position. Slowly stand up and push the dumbbell up over the head. Lower the weight as you return to squatting position. Repeat 8 to 12 times before lifting the left arm.

5 One Arm Row

Holding a dumbbell in the right hand, take one step back with the right leg into a lunge position. Slowly raise the dumbbell to your arm pit with the elbow pointing to the ceiling. Return dumbbell to starting position. Repeat 8 to 12 times before stepping back with the left leg and lifting the left arm.

6 Lateral Raise

Holding a dumbbell in the right hand with the palm facing the right shoulder, sit back into a squat position. Slowly stand up and swing the dumbbell up to the side until the elbow is parallel to the ground. Lower the weight as you return to squatting position. Repeat 8 to 12 times before lifting the left arm.

7 Biceps / Triceps Rock

Hold a dumbbell in each hand. As you rock to the left side, slowly curl the right hand toward the shoulder and extend the left arm behind the body. Now rock to the right side, curl the left hand toward the shoulder and extend the right arm behind the body. Repeat 8 to 12 times.

8 Two arm swing

Hold the ends of a dumbbell with both hands. Sit back into a squat position. Slowly stand up and swing the dumbbell up to shoulder level. Lower the weight as you return to squatting position. Repeat 8 to 12 times.

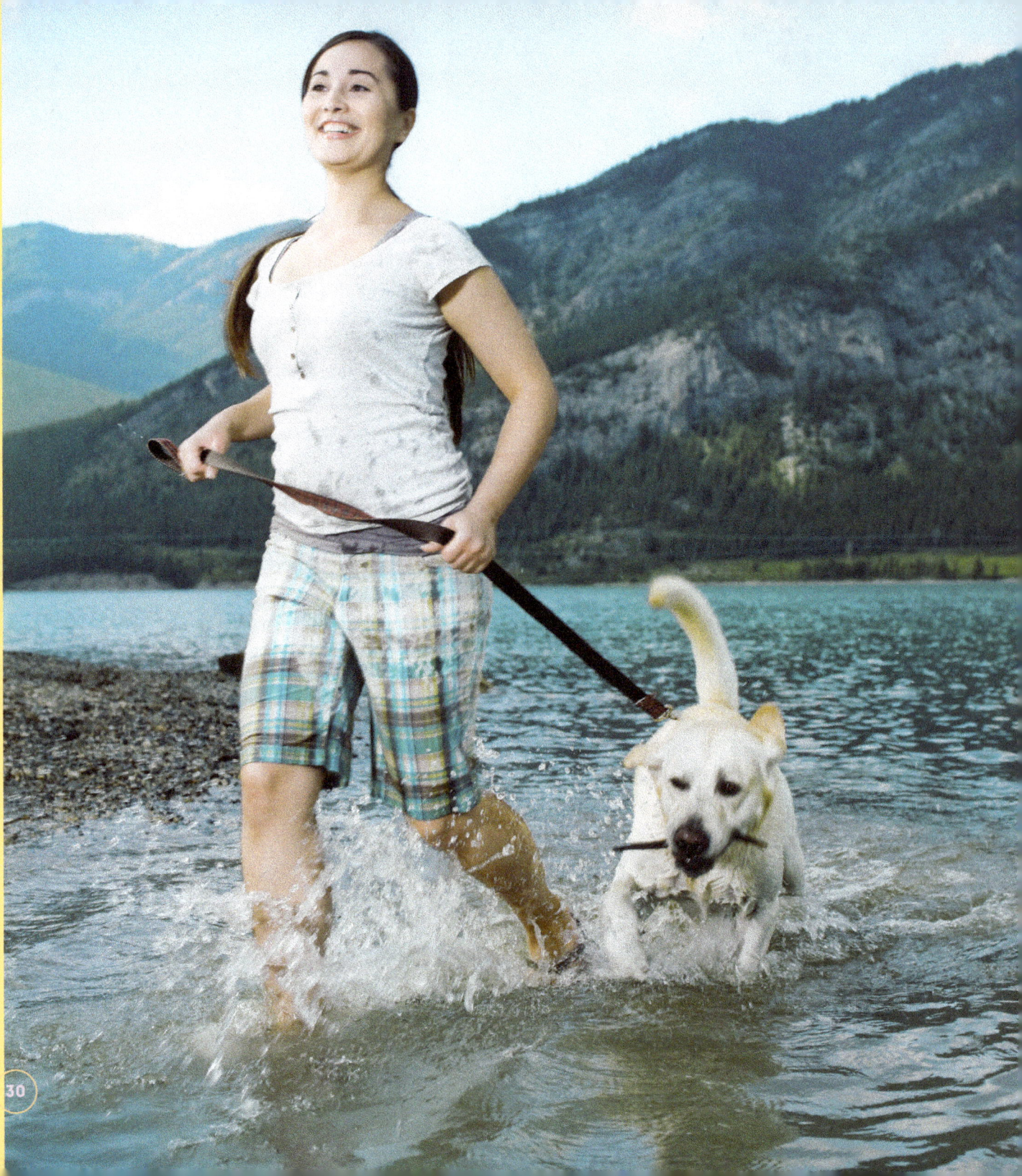

Conclusion

Walking your dog reaps more than the given health benefits. It provides you with empowerment to take control of your health, personal fulfillment, and well-being while creating a bond with your dog. If you don't own a dog, now might be the best time to go to the local shelter and adopt a dog. Or if your lifestyle is not conducive to owning a dog, volunteer to walk shelter dogs during the week. Either way everyone wins!

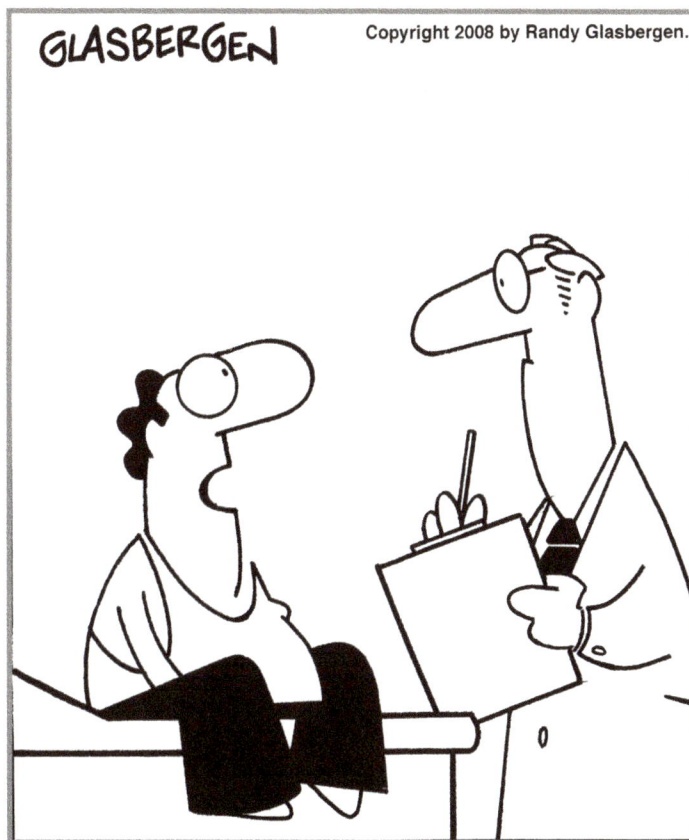

GLASBERGEN

Copyright 2008 by Randy Glasbergen.

"Eat less and exercise more? That's the most ridiculous fad diet I've heard of yet!"

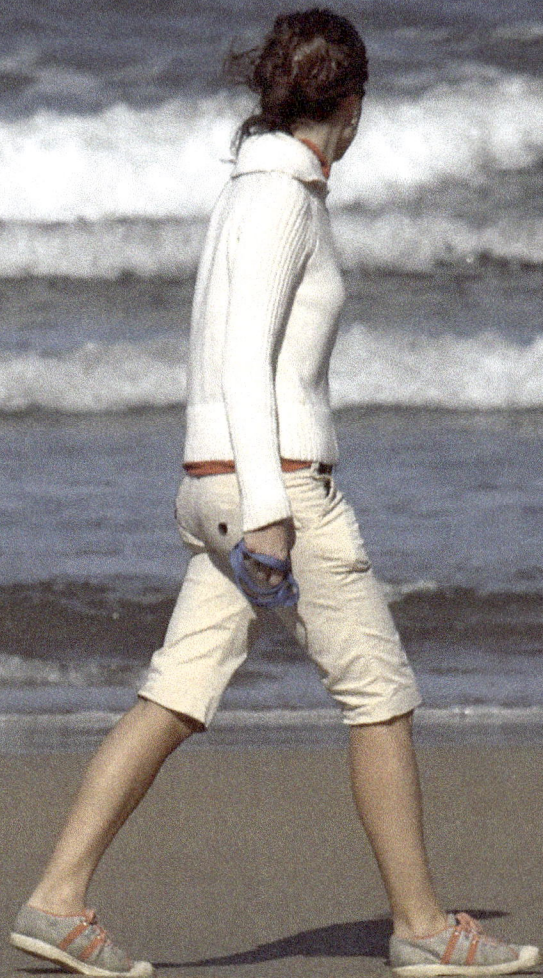
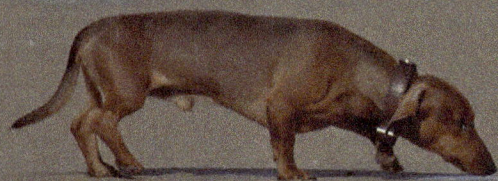

www.ingramcontent.com/pod-product-compliance
Lightning Source LLC
Chambersburg PA
CBHW080927050426

42334CB00055B/2834